Foreword

Firstly, thank you for picking up a copy of Vegan Baking for beginners. This guide will show you how to get started baking things as a new (or experienced) Vegan.

If you're BRAND NEW to being a Vegan, you might be feeling a bit confused. There are so many options and it's hard to know what to cook/eat or how to do it. That's why this guide was created. We have another book for Vegan smoothie recipes but this one is focused on baking and cooking substantial meals or snacks.

As the title suggests, this guide is also aimed at baking things that will have an effect on your brainpower. Our brains are probably the most important tool we have for achieving what we want in this short life, and for that reason it's so very important to give our brains what they need to thrive.

Often it comes down to having a wide variety of fruits and vegetables and making sure you have enough 'essential amino acids' but we'll get onto that a bit later. For now just know that this guide is aimed at helping you learn how to cook delicious vegan food, that will improve your body, health, and mind.

As you've probably picked up this was written by myself, an Entrepreneur, hence the focus on brain health and cognitive function. It's something that's always interested me and ever since I was a young man I have wanted to improve my brain and get my body and mind to perform as well as possible.

You may be familiar with the film 'Limitless' in which the protagonist takes a mystery pill which allows him to access all of his brainpower and achieve incredible things very quickly. I've always been obsessed with that idea, the idea that each of us can be so much more than we are.

And that's part of the reason for writing this book, because I truly believe that a Vegan diet can REALLY help you become a better person, both physically and mentally. Since going Vegan my brainpower has JUMPED up a huge amount and I've been able to do some awesome things.

One of the best ways THIS BOOK IS DIFFERENT from a lot of other baking guides and vegan cookbooks, is that I've tried (wherever possible) to not use the same old ingredients over and over again. Of course things like Oats and base ingredients are hard to NOT have in a recipe but even then, I've tried to find recipes that use a diverse range of ingredients.

This is so you don't get bored, AND so that your body gets a variety of foods which is very good for it! I've seen lots of cookbooks that just have loads of recipes with very similar ingredients. This book is not like that.

And that marks the end of my little rant and we'll now get onto the baking recipes. You can use them however you wish and form this point on, there's no 'order' to this book, you can choose which recipes you'd like to use (or not) as you wish.

I'll be back at the end of the book to talk a bit about how you can use the Vegan diet to improve yourself and give you some ideas for how to structure a basic meal plan for a week etc.

How to use these recipes

The recipes in the book are easy to make and not time-consuming at all. They are all created using vegan and nutritionally dense ingredients. Although the specifically chosen ingredients focus on enhancing the health and functioning of the brain, they also improve your overall health.

The recipes are free of toxins, GMO's, processed foods, artificial colours, and as we said, are totally vegan-friendly.

The recipes in the book are both bake and no-bake recipes, so they benefit both raw vegans, plant-based vegetarians and people who want to be mentally fit. All the recipes are designed to enhance your attention span, lift the brain fog, maintain brain health, and prevent mental illnesses.

Most of the recipes can be made in batches and stored for months. The bars, granola, energy balls are an excellent and healthy substitute for a snack or vitamin supplement.

If you don't have an ingredient

If you are allergic to any particular ingredient, then you can substitute them in the following ways.

1. If you don't have a specific type of meal/flour, then you can just buy the nuts or seeds and blend them to make the desired meal/flour. For instance, if the recipe calls for an almond meal then just blend some almonds in a blender to get the almond meal.

2. If you want to replace maple syrup, then you can add in the equal quantity of agave, molasses, coconut nectar, brown rice syrup.

3. If you wish to replace nuts with a different kind of nut, then maintain equal proportions while substituting. For instance, 1 cup of chopped almonds can be substituted by 1 cup of chopped walnuts/ cashews/ hazelnuts/ pecans.

Brain tonic Granola Recipe

This granola recipe is quick, tastes amazing, and you can use it to make granola bars or energy balls. The granola makes a super quick breakfast meal. You can add the granola to your favourite milk (almond/coconut/soy) and top it with your favourite fruits and berries.

You can eat it with coconut yogurt and fruits as a vegan parfait. Unlike other granolas, this recipe is specially curated with superfoods that benefit and uplift the brain health. So, let's begin baking it!

Servings – 7 servings

Baking time- 35 minutes

Ingredients list

Wet ingredients

Virgin coconut oil – ¼ cup

Maple syrup/agave syrup – ½ cup

Almond butter/peanut butter – 3tbsp.

Dry ingredients

Unsweetened Cocoa powder – ¼ cup

Rolled oats – 1 ½ cup

Instant oats – 1 ½ cup

Walnuts – ¼ cup (chopped)

Almonds – ¼ cup (chopped)

Cashews – ¼ cup (sliced in half)

Flaxseeds – 2 tbsp.

Chia seeds – ¼ cup

Cacao nibs – ¼ cup

Instructions

1. Preheat the oven to 300 degrees Fahrenheit.

2. Add all the wet ingredients in a microwave-safe bowl.

3. Place the bowl in the microwave for 30 seconds. It will melt the coconut oil and almond/peanut butter.

4. Mix all the wet ingredients thoroughly so that all the ingredients are combined. (keep the bowl in the microwave to prevent the coconut oil for re-freezing.)

5. In a large mixing bowl, add in all the dry ingredients in their specified ratio. If you want to substitute any nuts or seeds, then you can substitute them in the same proportion.

6. Mix the dry ingredients with the help of a spatula, so that the chia seeds and cocoa powder covers all the oats. At this point, the wet ingredients should look like a light brown mixture.

7. Pour in the wet mixture over the dry mix and combine the two. There should be no dry patches left.

8. Cover a large baking tray with parchment paper or a silicone baking mat.

9. Spread the mixture over the tray evenly with the help of a spatula.

10. Place the tray in the oven and bake for 25-30 minutes at 300 degrees.

11. Make sure to check the granola after 15 minutes; you can gently mix it to ensure that it is not burnt or undercooked from any side.

12. After 25-30 minutes, take out the tray and let the granola cool completely (2 hours).

13. You can transfer the granola to an airtight glass container and store it for months.

Nutritional insight

1. Virgin coconut oil – Coconut oil provides the brain with ketones (fuel for the brain) after it metabolizes. It is because it has MCT (medium chain triglycerides) which are good fats. The ketones in coconut oil can instantly cross the blood-brain barrier and provide energy for the brain.

2. Maple syrup – Maple syrup has a compound similar to resveratrol that is found in red wine. It helps in protecting the primary brain proteins beta-amyloid and tau peptide from clumping and folding. It can prevent the Alzheimer's disease by protecting these two proteins found in the brain cells.

3. Walnuts – The brain-shaped nut provides DHA to the brain which is a type of Omega 3 acid, vitamin E, and folate. It also helps in lowering bad cholesterol. Walnuts help in improving the cognitive functions, memory retention, and protect the brain from age-related problems.

4. Almonds – A great source of vitamin E, B6, Iron, calcium, magnesium and lean proteins. Almonds help in boosting memory, prevent free radical damage (vitamin E), and repairs brain cells.

5. Chia seeds – The chia seeds contain ALA (Alpha-linoleic acid), omega 3 fatty acids, antioxidants, 9 important amino acids and glucose. In brief, they provide all the fuel that is needed for the brain cells to function properly, and also prevents the brain from free radical damage (antioxidant).

6. Flax seeds – It is another rich source of ALA, and omega 3. The omega 3 helps the neurons to receive and send signals efficiently. It helps in improving the cognitive function of the brain.

7. Cashews – Cashew nuts have a high concentration of MUFA (mono saturated fatty acids), zinc, magnesium, iron, phosphorus, folate, vitamin K. The good fats in cashew provide fuel to the brain, the nutrients and minerals improve the synaptic transmission function, regulate the neurotransmitter pathways.

8. Cacao Nibs – They are rich in poly
   phenols, flavanols, magnesium, copper,
   iron, and proteins. They help the brain by
   increasing the blood flow and the cognitive
   functions of the brain. Polyphenols help
   the brain by reducing toxicity, and
   inflammation. Copper is responsible for
   the proper functioning of enzymes in the
   brain and its deficiency results in mental
   illnesses.

9. Oats – Oats are the best meal for the brain
   because it fulfils glucose and fat
   requirements of the brain. The sugar in
   oats is released steadily (low on the
   glycemic index) and provides a continuous
   supply of glucose to the brain. Oats are
   rich in good fats such as Omega 3 and
   Omega 6 fatty acid; these fats help in
   reducing cholesterol and promote brain
   health.

Vitamins such as A, C, K, B6, and thiamine are also present in oats. Important elements that are required for nerve functions, synaptic functions, neurotransmitter synthesis, enzyme synthesis such as Zinc, copper, selenium, iron, manganese, magnesium, potassium, phosphorus, and sodium are also present in good quantity in oats.

Crunchy granola bar

A quick bake recipe that makes a breakfast bar.

Prep time – 10 minutes

Bake time – 30 minutes

Ingredient list

Roasted Oats – 1 cup

Roasted Almonds – ½ cup

Roasted Peanuts – ½ cup

Pumpkin seeds – ¼ cup

Chia seeds – ¼ cup

Almond butter – ½ cup

Maple syrup – 4 tbsp (add more if needed)

Coconut oil – 4 tbsp

Himalayan pink salt – 1 tsp

Water – 3 tbsp

Instructions

1. Preheat the oven to 350 F.

2. To make the sauce, add coconut oil, almond butter, maple syrup, Himalayan salt, water in a saucepan. Place the saucepan on low heat and mix until everything melts and forms a thick sauce.

3. Transfer the sauce to a large mixing bowl and add roasted oats, peanuts, almonds, chia seeds, pumpkin seeds to it.

4. Mix the sauce and the dry ingredients. The mixture should look slightly wet and dough-like.

5. Transfer the mixture to a baking pan lined with parchment paper.

6. Bake at 350 F for 30 minutes.

7. Let it cool completely and then cut the bars as per your requirements.

BOCA Baked bars

The name is the acronym for the main ingredients in the bars. This recipe is easy, delicious, and chewy.

Prep time – 10 minutes

Bake time – 20 - 25 minutes

Oven settings – 300 F (150 C)

Ingredient list

1. Ripe Bananas – 2 large (riper the better)
2. Raw cacao powder – 1/4 cup (add 3 tbsp for a milder flavour)
3. Coconut oil – 1 tbsp
4. Rolled oats – 1 cup
5. Cacao nibs – 2 tbsp
6. Chopped almonds – 2 tbsp
7. Shredded dry coconut – 1/2 cup
8. Raisins – 10 – 13 (can be omitted)

9. Maple syrup – 2 tbsp (as per taste)

Instructions

1. Preheat the oven to 300 F.

2. Begin by mashing the ripe bananas in a bowl. Mash them until no lumps remain.

3. Add the coconut oil, cacao powder, oats, chopped almonds, shredded coconut, raisins to the mashed bananas. Mix all the ingredients until everything is combined.

4. Taste the mixture to check the sweetness and add the desired amount of maple syrup to the mixture. Keep in mind that after baking, the sweetness decreases a bit, so make the mixture slightly sweeter than you'd prefer.

5. Line a baking tray with parchment paper.

6. Take 2 tablespoons of the mixture and mold it into the shape of a bar. Place it on the baking tray. Repeat the step for the rest of the bars.

7. Keep some space between the bars so that they don't stick to each other.

8. Bake for 20- 25 minutes. Check the bars
    after 20 minutes so that they don't burn
    (every oven is a bit different).

9. The bars are chewy and dense so don't
    wait long for the bars to be crunchy as you
    might overcook them.

Nutritional benefits

1. Bananas – They release glucose slowly
    into the bloodstream which is a perfect
    fuel for the brain. Bananas are a rich
    source of magnesium which reduces
    ammonia toxicity in the brain. It contains
    vitamin B6 and folate which help in
    preventing brain from degenerative
    diseases. They contain vitamins and
    minerals such as zinc, copper, phosphorus,
    potassium, vitamin K, vitamin E which are
    responsible for maintaining electrical
    signals, synaptic functions,
    neurotransmitter synthesis, and
    regulation.

2. Oats, almonds, coconut oil, cacao nibs, maple syrup - Oats fulfil the glucose and fat requirements of your brain. The sugar in oats is released steadily (low on the glycemic index) and provides a continuous supply of glucose to the brain. Oats are rich in good fats such as Omega 3 and Omega 6 fatty acid; these fats help in reducing cholesterol and promote brain health.

Vitamins such as A, C, K, B6, and thiamine are also present in oats. Important elements that are required for nerve functions, synaptic functions, neurotransmitter synthesis, enzyme synthesis such as Zinc, copper, selenium, iron, manganese, magnesium, potassium, phosphorus, and sodium are also present in good quantity in oats.

Fruity granola bar

This Fruity granola bar is light and tasty snack. It can be stored for months in a glass container, in a cool place. If you are allergic to nuts then, it is a perfect alternative to nutty granola bars.

Prep time – 10 minutes

Ingredients list

1. Chopped dried apples – ½ cup
2. Chopped Mangoes – ½ cup
3. Dried apricots – ½ cup
4. Dried cranberries – ¼ cup
5. Coconut flakes – ¼ cup
6. Old fashioned oats – ½ cup
7. Maple syrup – 4 tbsp
8. Virgin frozen Coconut oil – ¼ cup
9. Himalayan pink salt – 2 tsp

Instructions

1. Add the apricots and oats to a blender and blend them for a minute or two.

2. In a small bowl add coconut oil, maple syrup, Himalayan pink salt. Place the bowl in the microwave for 30 seconds (you can heat the mixture over the stove on low heat). This mixture is the 'sauce' of the granola bars.

3. In a large mixing bowl add the chopped dried apples, chopped dried mangoes, dried cranberries, coconut flakes. With the help of a spatula mix all the ingredients well.

4. Add the microwaved sauce, blended apricots to the mixing bowl and with the mix well with a spatula or your hands.

5. You can add a tablespoon of melted coconut oil and maple syrup, if the mixture is a little dry.

6. After, the mixture attains a dough like consistency, place the mixture into a baking tray lined with parchment paper. Pat down and flatten the mixture on the baking tray. Maintain the thickness of an inch or so, and place the baking tray into the freezer for an hour to set.

7. When the bars are set firmly, cut them into the desired size and enjoy.

Nutrition list

1. Mango – They provide antioxidant to the brain that helps in fighting free radical damage. Vitamin B6 found in mangoes is responsible for the synthesis of neurotransmitters and aids in nerve impulse transfer. Vitamin A provides retinol to the brain which is linked to neurogenesis. Mangoes are also rich in glutamine, copper, folate and potassium that help in maintaining brain health.

2. Apples – Apples boost the production of acetylcholine which helps the electric signal transfer in the synapse (neuron to neuron). Apples also contains all the vital trace elements required for optimum brain health.

3. Apricots – Apricots are a rich source of potassium which is responsible for increasing attention span, reducing brain fog and aids in oxygen supply to the brain. They also contain vitamin B6, magnesium that helps in neurotransmitter generation and in nerve impulse generation respectively.

4. Cranberries – They contain ursolic acid which is known to reverse cognitive damage and is also linked with preventing degenerative diseases.

5. Oats, coconut oil/flakes, maple syrup - Oats fulfil the glucose and fat requirements of your brain. The sugar in oats is released steadily (low on the glycemic index) and provides a continuous supply of glucose to the brain. Oats are rich in good fats such as Omega 3 and Omega 6 fatty acid; these fats help in reducing cholesterol and promote brain health.

Vitamins such as A, C, K, B6, and thiamine are also present in oats. Important elements that are required for nerve functions, synaptic functions, neurotransmitter synthesis, enzyme synthesis such as Zinc, copper, selenium, iron, manganese, magnesium, potassium, phosphorus, and sodium are also present in good quantity in oats.

Cashew and date bars

Cashew and date bars taste creamy and are easy to make. The recipe can be made into both vegan bars and energy balls.

Prep time – 10 minutes

Ingredients list

1. Cashew flour – 3/4 cup
2. Pitted Medjool dates – 20
3. Himalayan pink salt – a pinch
4. Slithered Almonds – 3 tbsp cup
5. Chia seeds – 3 tbsp

Instructions

1. If you don't have cashew flour, then add the dried cashews in a blender (ideally a powerful blunderer seed grinder) and blend them for a minute or so until you have a find powder.

2. In a blender, add the Medjool dates, a pinch of Himalayan pink salt and blend them until you achieve a dough like consistency. IMPORTANT: Use soft medjool dates and NOT dried dates. If you try and blend dried dates you'll ruin your blender.

3. Transfer the blended dates into a mixing bowl. Add the cashew flour, almonds, chia seeds to the mixing bowl. Mix the ingredients until they are all incorporated well.

4. if you want to make granola bars, transfer the mixture to a pan or a baking tray covered with parchment paper. With the back of a spoon flatten the mixture evenly on the tray. Place it in the freezer for an hour and cut into small pieces.

5. If you wish to make the mixture into energy balls, then roll the mixture into medium sized balls and store them in the refrigerator.

Nutrition list

1. Medjool dates – Dates contain a very high amount of sugar but, since they have a low glycamic rating, they are good for the brain. The dates provide a continuous supply of glucose to the brain which provides better focus. It also contains magnesium, manganese, vitamin B6, copper, zinc, potassium, phosphorus which help the brain by preventing degenerative diseases and support vital brain functions.

2. Almonds, cashews, chia seeds – Mentioned previously

Carrot cake bars

These bats taste just like a carrot cake but are healthier and quicker to make than most bars. No baking required for this one!

Prep time – 10 minutes

Ingredients list

1. Shredded carrots – 1 cup
2. Raisins – 2 tbsp
3. Walnuts – ½ cup
4. Pecans – ½ cup
5. Pitted Medjool dates – ½ cup
6. Almond butter – ¼ cup
7. Maple syrup – 2 tbsp
8. Oats – ½ cup

Instructions

1. In a blender add dates, oats, pecans and blend for a minute.

2. In a small bowl add almond butter, maple syrup and microwave it for 30 seconds. Take it out of the microwave and mix the ingredients (referred to as sauce).

3. Transfer the contents of the blender and the sauce to a large mixing bowl. Mix in the carrots, walnuts, and raisins. You can use your hands to mix the ingredients well.

4. Once the mixture forms a dough-like consistency transfer it on a parchment lined baking tray.

5. Press the mixture firmly on to the baking tray with the help of a spoon.

6. Place the tray in the refrigerator and let it cool for 1 hour.

7. After an hour your can check if the mixture has set, if not give it 20 more minutes in the freezer.

8. Cut the mixture into the desirable size and enjoy.

Nutritional benefits

1. Carrots – The carrots contain luteolin which helps in decreasing age-related inflammation and memory decline. They are a rich source of vitamin A, vitamin C, iron, Calcium, Magnesium, vitamin B6. The tryptophan in the carrots helps you feel calm and stress-free. The beta-carotene in the carrots is a powerful antioxidant, that helps in fighting free radical damage. Carrots have proved effective in preventing Alzheimer's and improving the cognitive functions.

2. Pecans – They hold the title of superfood for the brain as they contain manganese which is important for the brains synaptic process. Copper and thiamine help in improving brain health by decreasing free radical damage and improving learning ability. They also contain choline, zinc, iron, vitamin B, vitamin C.

3. Raisins – They provide glucose to the brain and also contain boron which is responsible for improving muscle and nerve functions (hand-eye coordination).

4. Medjool dates – Mentioned previously

3. Walnuts, oats, maple syrup, almonds -
   Mentioned previously

Dense dark forest bars

The dense forest bars are chocolaty, sweet, and crunchy. The bars need to be stored in the fridge or freezer as the main component is chocolate.

Prep time – 15 minutes

Ingredients list

1. Dark chocolate (chopped) – 2 cups
2. Agave syrup/ maple syrup – 2 to 3 tbsp
3. Pistachios split in half – 1/2 cup
4. Almonds split in half – 1/4 cup
5. Chopped hazelnuts – ¼ cup
6. Puffed rice – ½ cup
7. Coconut oil - ¼ cup
8. Himalayan salt - pinch

Instructions

1. Keep a sauce pan on low heat and melt coconut oil in the saucepan. Once the coconut oil melts, add the chopped dark chocolate, Himalayan salt in the pan, and keep stirring. Ensure the heat is low and the chocolate doesn't burn.

2. Once the chocolate and the coconut oil melt completely (forms a chocolate sauce), take the pan off the stove. Add the maple syrup and mix. If you are happy with the sweetness, you can omit or add less maple syrup.

3. In a bowl add in the pistachios, hazelnuts, almonds, puffed rice and mix.

4. The next step is to create three layers two layers of chocolate, one on top and bottom with a middle layer of nut mixture.

5. In a baking pan (9x9) lined with parchment paper pour half dark chocolate sauce evenly. On top of the chocolate layer sprinkle the dry mixture evenly. Pour a layer of the leftover chocolate sauce so that it appears like a sandwich.

6. Place the pan in the freezer for an hour to allow the chocolate set completely.

Nutritional benefits

1. Pistachio – The green nut has a higher content of monosaturated fatty acids, vitamin A, vitamin C, vitamin B6, calcium, potassium, sodium, phosphorus, selenium, iron, copper, zinc, and magnesium. Pistachio prevents the brain cells from inflammation, provides antioxidants to fight free radical damage, supports mental alertness and cognitive function of the brain.

2. Dark chocolate – The dark chocolate is a source of great brain food. It contains flavanols that help in increasing blood flow to the brain. It contains vitamin B12, which is important for nerve health. It also contains calcium, antioxidants, copper, selenium, zinc, manganese, sodium, Phosphorus, magnesium, potassium, and iron. Dark chocolate helps in improving working memory, prevents mental decline.

3. Hazelnuts – They are a rich source of good
   fat, folate, vitamin E, B6, C,
   proanthocyanins, quercetins, flavonoids. It
   helps in increasing brains cognitive
   functions and improves brain health.
   Thiamine helps in maintaining a healthy
   nerve function. The high level of vitamin E
   (Tocopherol) prevents the brain from
   diseases such as Alzheimer's, dementia,
   Parkinson's.

4. Coconut oil and almonds – Mentioned
   previously

Sesame balls

You will be surprised how good these energy balls taste. Especially, if you have never tried sesame seeds.

Prep time – 10 minutes

Ingredient list

1. Roasted sesame seeds - 2 cups

2. Medjool dates – 3/4 cup (pitted)

3. Coconut oil – 1 tbsp

4.

Instructions

1. Add the pitted Medjool dates, roasted sesame seeds, coconut oil to a blender and blend for 1 minutes or until everything combines and forms a dough.

2. Begin rolling the dough into bite-sized balls.

3. Store them in a cool dry place or in the refrigerator.

Nutritional Benefits

1. Sesame seeds – They are a rich source of iron, magnesium, zinc, potassium, phosphorus, and selenium. The rich mineral content helps to maintain brains health and improves cognitive functioning. Sesame seeds contain a high amount of copper which is essential for preventing the brain from degenerative diseases such a dementia, Alzheimer's.

2. Medjool dates - Mentioned previously

3. Coconut oil - Mentioned previously

Green Matcha Balls

The green matcha balls are vibrant, full of nutrients and filled with energy. You can store them in the freezer and they can last up to 4 days, if kept in the refrigerator.

Prep time – 15 minutes

Ingredients list

1. Matcha – 1 tbsp

2. Water – 3 tbsp

3. Ripe avocado – 1 cup

4. Shredded Coconut – ¼ cup

5. Vanilla – 1 tsp

6. Soaked cashews – ½ cup

7. Almond meal – ½ cup

8. Maple syrup – 4 tbsp (as per your taste)

9. Himalayan salt – pinch

Instructions

1. In a small bowl add 1 tablespoon of matcha powder and 3 tablespoons of water so that the matcha powder dissolves completely.

2. Add the soaked cashews to a blender and blend them for a minute or two, until they form a wet, pastey sort of mixture. You can also add 2 tablespoons of water if the paste is too thick.

3. In a large mixing bowl, mash the ripe avocado so that no lumps remain.

4. Add the blended cashew paste, matcha solution, almond meal, vanilla, maple syrup, Himalayan salt to the mashed avocado.

5. With the help of a spatula mix all the ingredients until you achieve a dough like consistency. If the dough seems too wet at this point, you can add a few more spoons of almond meal to achieve the desired consistency.

6. Divide the dough into equal proportions and roll them into bite-size balls.

7. In a plate spread the shredded coconut and roll the balls on the plate to get an even coating of coconut.

8. Store in a cool, dry place.

Nutrition benefits

1. Matcha – It contains l-theanine which is helps in improving memory and learning benefits. L-theanine provides calmness to the brain without any side-effects that caffeine has. It contains a high content of antioxidants that prevent the brain from free radical damage. The unique vitamin and mineral content of matcha helps the brain to boost brain cell production. It also contains vitamins A, vitamin C, potassium, EGCG. Epigallocatechin gallate helps the brain by enhancing memory retention, prevents mental illnesses, and increases the attention span.

2. Avocado – It is a rich source of monosaturated fats aka the good fat, omega 3 and omega 6 fatty acids. The good fats and omega acids are the fuel to the brain and help in maintaining the good health of the brain. Avocados are a rich source of vitamins and minerals, as they contain 20 minerals and vitamins. It contains vitamins A, C, E, K, B6 and riboflavin, choline, folate, niacin, thiamine. Avocados improve the blood flow to the brain and the body resulting in better functioning and enhancing cognitive abilities of the brain.

3. Almond, cashew, maple syrup, coconut – Mentioned previously

Figates Energy Balls

If you feel hungry and fatigued most of the times, even if you eat a lot, then these are perfect for you. These energy balls can be stored up to 2 months (that is if you don't devour them sooner). If you don't have a sweet tooth then, I would advise you to add less Medjool dates.

Prep time – 10 minutes

Ingredients list

1. Dried figs – 3/4 cup

2. Medjool dates (pitted) – ½ cup

3. Oat flour – ¼ cup

4. Almond meal – ¼ cup

5. Vanilla – 1tsp (can be omitted)

6. Desiccated coconut – ¼ cup

7. Coconut oil – 2 tbsp

8. Himalayan salt – pinch

Instructions

1. Add the dried figs and Medjool dates to the blender and blend for a minute. The blended mixture should be dough like.

2. Continue to add oat flour, almond meal, coconut oil, desiccated coconut, vanilla, Himalayan salt to the dates and fig mixture in the blender.

3. Blend it for a minute or until everything combines well.

4. Take out the mixture from the blender and roll the dough into bite size balls.

Nutritional benefits

1. Dried figs – Figs provide natural glucose to the brain which is its primary fuel. They contain a high amount of potassium which is responsible for basic brain functioning. Potassium helps in generating an action potential which is required to transfer electric signals from one neuron to the other. Figs are also a good source of vitamin B6 which is a primary component used for the synthesis of neurotransmitters. Manganese helps the brain by converting glutamate to glutamine and reduces the glutamate toxicity. Figs also contain selenium, zinc, copper, iron, calcium that contributes to a healthy brain.

2. Medjool dates – Mentioned previously

3. Almond meal, coconut, oats - Mentioned previously

Choco-nut balls

A sweet, filling, and healthy recipe for every occasion.

Prep time – 10 minutes

Ingredient list

Desiccated coconut – 2 cups

Grated Dark chocolate – 1 ½ cup

Vanilla – 1 tbsp

Maple syrup – 3 tbsp (add more if needed)

Instructions

1. Add the grated dark chocolate, desiccated coconut, maple syrup to a microwave safe bowl and microwave it for 30 seconds.

2. Add the vanilla to the mixture and mix it with the help of a spatula until the mixture begins to look dough-like.

3. Roll the dough into small balls and enjoy.

Nutritional benefits

1. Coconut, maple syrup – Mentioned previously

2. Dark chocolate - Mentioned previously

Choco-hazelnut balls

This recipe is one of my all-time favourites as it suffices my cravings for Nutella. The recipe is healthy, free of any toxic ingredient and tastes amazing.

Prep time – 10 minutes

Ingredient list

1. Cacao nibs – 2 tbsp

2. Hazelnut meal – 1 cup (blended hazelnuts)

3. Chopped Hazelnut – ¼ cup

4. Dark chocolate – ¾ cup

5. Coconut oil – 3 tbsp

6. Maple syrup – 2 tbsp

7. Himalayan salt – pinch

Instructions

1. In a microwave safe bowl add the chopped dark chocolate, coconut oil, maple syrup, Himalayan salt and microwave it for 30 seconds. Stir the mixture and microwave it again for 10 seconds. You can heat it on a low heat as well.

2. Once the chocolate melts completely, you can transfer it to a large bowl.

3. Add the hazelnut meal (blended hazelnut), chopped hazelnuts, and cacao nibs to the bowl.

4. Mix all the ingredients in the bowl with the help of a spatula until everything combines well.

5. Let the mixture cool for a few minutes.

6. When the mixture has cooled slightly, you can roll the mixture into bite-sized balls.

7. You can store the Choco-hazelnut ball in the refrigerator for up to a month.

Nutritional benefits

1. Hazelnut, dark chocolate– Mentioned previously

2. Coconut oil, cacao nibs, maple syrup - Mentioned previously

Chocolate peanut energy balls

The recipe makes delicious energy balls that taste similar to snickers and are healthier.

Prep time – 10 minutes

Ingredient list

Roasted peanuts – 1 cup

Roasted cashews – 1 cup

Cocoa powder – 2 tbsp

Dark chocolate – ½ cup (chopped)

Coconut oil – 3 tbsp

Peanut butter – 3 tbsp

Himalayan pink salt – 1 tsp

Maple syrup – 3 tbsp (add according to taste)

Instructions

1. In a microwave safe bowl add the chopped dark chocolate, cocoa powder, coconut oil, peanut butter, maple syrup, Himalayan salt and microwave it for 30 seconds. Stir the mixture and microwave it again for 10 seconds. You can heat it on a low flame as well.

2. Once all the ingredients melt and form a thick sauce, transfer it to a large bowl.

3. Add roasted peanuts and cashews in the blender and blend them finely. Once the peanuts and cashews are blended transfer them to the bowl containing the chocolate sauce.

4. Mix all the ingredients in the bowl with the help of a spatula until everything combines well.

5. You can roll the mixture into bite-sized balls and enjoy them at any time of the day.

Nutritional benefits

1. Peanuts – Peanuts are a rich source of fat that is the basic fuel for the brain. It also contains vitamin E, Vitamin B6 which prevent free radical damage and in the synthesis of neurotransmitter. They are rich in copper, iron, zinc, magnesium which helps in generating the action potential, prevent degenerative diseases.

2. Cashews, maple syrup, coconut oil – Mentioned previously

3. Dark chocolate - Mentioned previously

Dates walnut matcha cake

Date-walnut-matcha cake is a perfect vegan dessert that is guiltfree, nutritionally dense, vibrant to look at, and of course, delicious.

Prep time – 10 minutes

Refrigerate for – 12 hours (overnight)

Ingredient list

1. Coconut cream- 1 ¼ cup
2. Matcha powder- 2 tbsp
3. Water – 3 tbsp
4. Pumpkin seeds – 2 tbsp
5. Pistachios – 2 tbsp
6. Dates pitted – 1 cup
7. Walnuts – ½ cup
8. Maple syrup – 2 tbsp (as per taste)
9. Ripe avocado mashed – 1/2 cup

Instructions

1. In a blender add pitted dates, walnuts and blend until everything is combined.

2. Take a cheesecake pan (springform pan) and evenly layer the dates and walnut blended mixture. Press the mixture firmly to create the even layer. Place it in the refrigerator while you make the second layer.

3. For the second layer, begin by dissolving 2 tbsp of matcha powder in 3tbsp water.

4. In a mixing bowl add in the coconut cream, matcha water, mashed avocado and whisk until everything is combined.

5. Add maple syrup to the above mixture and check the sweetness. You can add more sweetener if 2 tbsp isn't enough.

6. Take out the cheesecake pan from the refrigerator and pour the creamy green mixture on top of the first layer.

7. Tap the cheesecake pan gently to get rid of any air bubbles.

8. Place the pan in the refrigerator for at least 12 hours.

9. When the coconut cream has set completely, garnish the top with chopped pistachios, and pumpkin seeds.

Nutritional benefits

1. Pumpkin seeds – These tiny seeds contain a high amount of Omega-3 and Omega-6 fatty acids which are vital for the brain to function. They are also rich in Vitamin A, C, K, B6, folate, and elements such as zinc, copper, magnesium, manganese, iron, sodium, potassium, phosphorus which help in neurotransmitter synthesis, enzyme synthesis. Pumpkin seeds also help in decreasing the brain fog due to their rich vitamin and mineral content.

2. Coconut, walnuts, maple syrup – Mentioned previously

3. Matcha and avocado – Mentioned previously

4. Pistachios – Mentioned previously

5. Medjool dates - Mentioned previously

Carrot cake

The recipe is a no-bake recipe and still delivers a rich and dense cake. It is slightly more time consuming than the other recipes, but it is worth it.

Prep time – 30 minutes

Refrigerate – 12 hours

Ingredient list
1. Medjool dates – 1 cup

2. Shredded carrots – 1cup

3. Coconut oil – 1 tbsp

4. Coconut cream – 1 cup

5. Cardamom powder – 1 tbsp

6. Chopped almonds – 2 tbsp

7. Maple syrup – 2 tbsp

8. Raisins – 10 - 13

Instructions

1. In a pan add 1 tbsp of coconut oil, and place it on the stove on low heat.

2. When the oil has melted completely, add in the shredded carrots, and sauté them for 2 minutes. Cover the pan with a lid, let the carrots cook for about 5 minutes on low flame.

3. After 5 minutes turn off the heat and add 2 to 3 tbsp of maples syrup to the carrots. Make sure to add maple syrup as per your taste.

4. Keep the carrot mixture on the side to cool down completely.

5. In a blender add the pitted dates and blend it for a minute or so.

6. Spread the dates on the cheesecake pan evenly. Place the pan in the refrigerator while you work on the filling.

7. Before you start working on the filling make sure the carrot mixture has cooled down completely. If the carrots haven't cooled yet, you can place the mixture in the freezer to cool.

8. Once the carrots have cooled down, transfer them into a mixing bowl.

9. Add coconut cream, cardamom powder, raisins into the bowl and whisk all the ingredients.

10. Take out the cheesecake pan from the refrigerator, and pour the carrot cream mixture on top of it.

11. Tap the tin gently to get rid of any air pockets, and place it in the refrigerator for at least 12 hours.

12. When the filling (carrot cream) has set completely add chopped almonds on top and enjoy.

Nutritional benefits

1. Cardamom powder – It is a rich source of antioxidants, potassium, phosphorus, magnesium, manganese, zinc, omega-3 and omega-6 fatty acid. It helps by preventing the brain from free radical damage and has been known to improve cognitive functions.

2. Carrots, Medjool dates, raisins, almonds, maple syrup – Mentioned previously

3. Coconut - Mentioned previously

How to make a diet plan

I'm going to write this section a bit differently than you're expecting. You're probably expecting a detailed diet plan showing you exactly what to eat and what not to eat. That's not how we're going to do this.

In layman terms, with a Vegan diet, the most important thing is that you get a lot of DIFFERENT foods, and that you get most of your calories from fruits, vegetables and legumes. The ingredients we've used in most of our recipes are perfect for brain health, and specifically, energy.

As long as you eat LOTS of greens, and use these recipes for brain boosts and energy bursts, you'll be a very healthy person. What I personally do it break down the day into four main sections..

Mornings: This is where we're at our most vulnerable and need to be rehydrated the most so here I drink a pint of cold filtered water, take my multivitamins and have a green smoothie consisting of several fruits, flax seeds, chia seeds, creatine, and spinach. I might sometimes have some rolled oats about an hour after this depending on what I'm doing or if I need more energy.

Middle of the day: A main meal that I would have prepared days before, in bulk. For example a Vegan shepherds pie or curry that I've prepared before, and either frozen of refrigerated in tubs. This is the cheapest and easiest way to eat during the day as a vegan!

Any snacks during the day: For my snacks I'll either eat nuts and seeds on their own, or I'll make one of the recipes in this book and cook up a big batch, and then snack on it throughout the week in the day times.

Evening meal: The evening meal will be another meal prepped sort of thing that I've cooked before and stored in tubs for the week. For example, a rice dish with lots of veg and herbs, or a salad. I don't like to have a heavy meal before bed as I find it stops me being able to sleep as well.

With every meal I have lots of fresh veg if I can, and in between all food I always drink filtered water. I don't drink anything sugary, and whenever I have a sweet snack it's always one mixed with some sort of slow releasee energy like a protein or a carb that is low on the glycol index. This prevents blood sugar problems and makes sure I don't have any sugar crashes.

And that's pretty much it! It really doesn't have to be complicated and in fact when you know what you can eat, and how to cook it, vegan eating becomes a lot easier than normal eating. Because you're not cooking any meat, it's also a lot easier and safer to prep food days before and just reheat or defrost it and eat it. This saves a lot of money and time.

As you can see, being a vegan actually works out a lot cheaper and easier despite what many people think!

Final words

And we've now come to the end of the recipes. Hopefully you've got a better idea of how you can eat and snack as a vegan, and what things are good for your brain health. These recipes are my best and the ones I actually use from week to week, so I'm sure you'll enjoy them as much as I do! Of course you can feel free to change them, add other ingredients as you see fit etc.

Free bonus and offers for my book readers: SECRET PAGE!

It's not quite over yet though, We've come to the end of this book but if you'd like to get a few free bonuses and interesting PDF downloads, head on over to this secret page on my website only for my book readers:

http://www.TranscendYourLimits.com/Bonus

Disclaimer

By reading this book you accept that you have full responsibility for any foods or drinks you do or do not consume, and you acknowledge that this book is NOT intended as professional medical advice or instructions. This is a collection of ideas, tips and recipes for smoothies for informational purposes.

Before changing your diet of consuming anything different, consult with your GP or physician who ill be able to instruct you further. By reading this you accept full responsibility for your health and what you do or do not consume.

Copyright